Blood Sugar Tracker

~weekly set up to track daily readings
~ includes images to color for your enjoyment

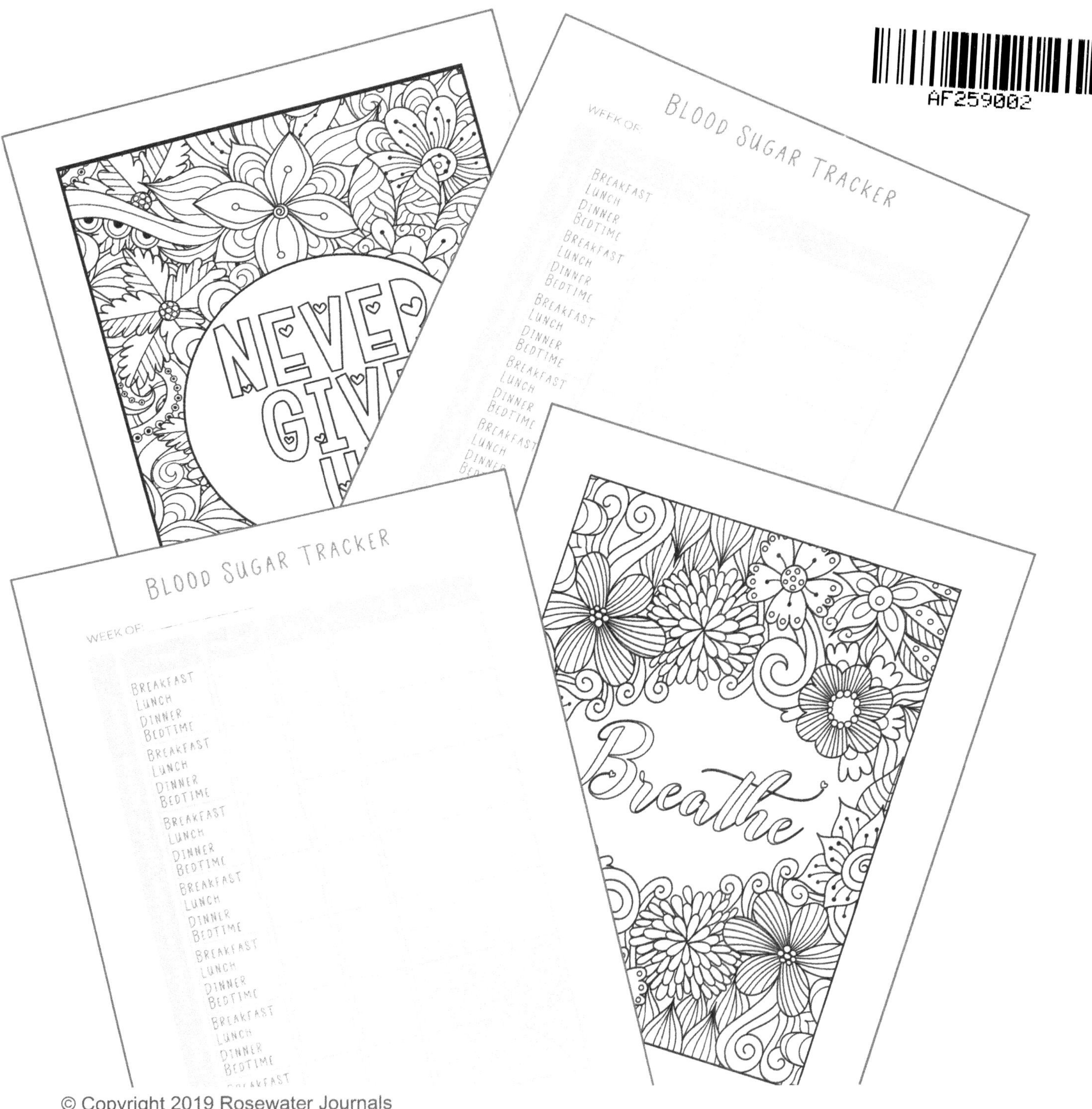

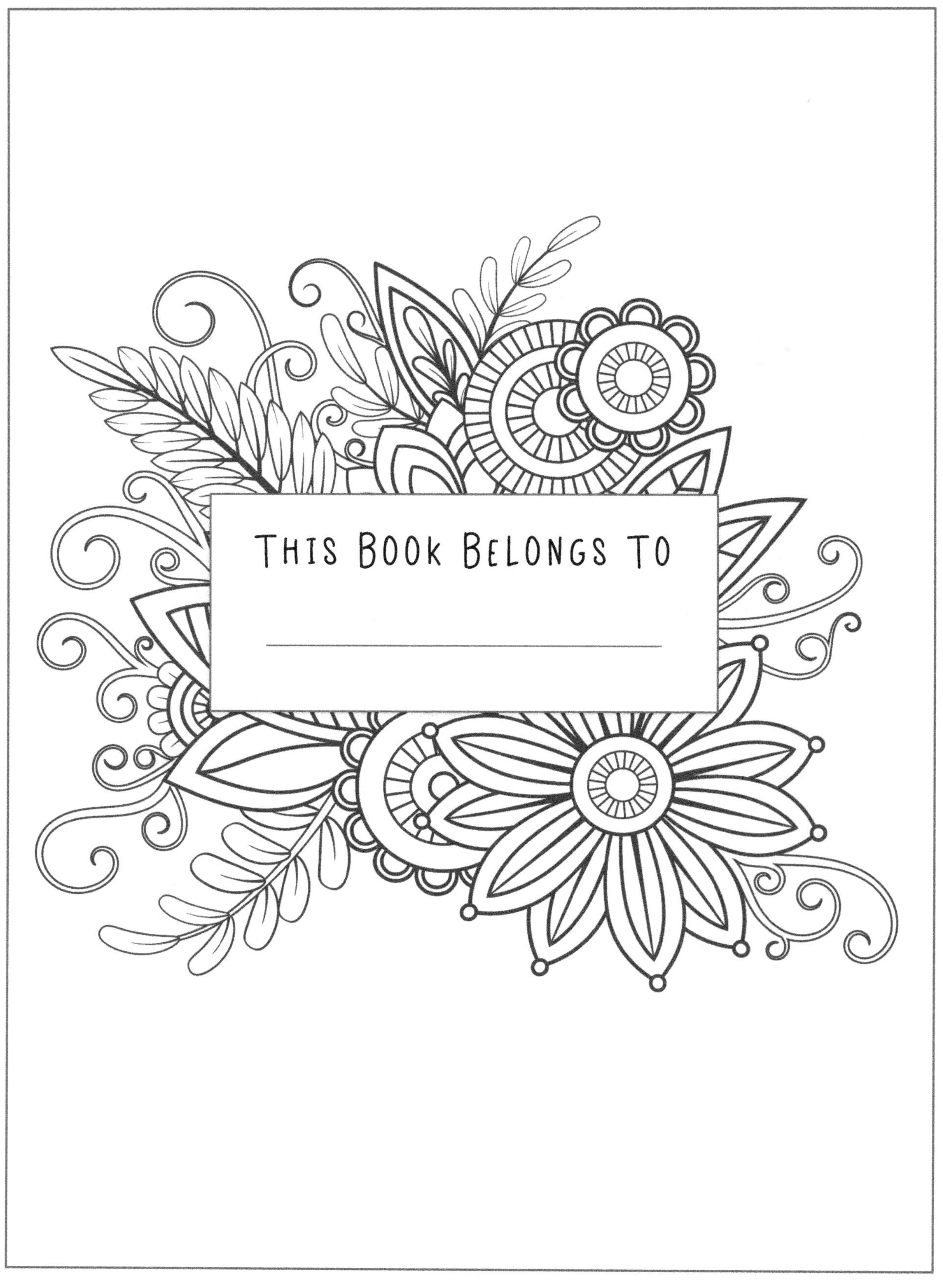

This Book Belongs To

Blood Sugar Tracker

WEEK OF: ______________________

BREAKFAST			
LUNCH			
DINNER			
BEDTIME			
BREAKFAST			
LUNCH			
DINNER			
BEDTIME			
BREAKFAST			
LUNCH			
DINNER			
BEDTIME			
BREAKFAST			
LUNCH			
DINNER			
BEDTIME			
BREAKFAST			
LUNCH			
DINNER			
BEDTIME			
BREAKFAST			
LUNCH			
DINNER			
BEDTIME			
BREAKFAST			
LUNCH			
DINNER			
BEDTIME			

Blood Sugar Tracker

WEEK OF: _________________________

	Time	Before	After	Notes
Sunday	Breakfast			
	Lunch			
	Dinner			
	Bedtime			
Monday	Breakfast			
	Lunch			
	Dinner			
	Bedtime			
Tuesday	Breakfast			
	Lunch			
	Dinner			
	Bedtime			
Wednesday	Breakfast			
	Lunch			
	Dinner			
	Bedtime			
Thursday	Breakfast			
	Lunch			
	Dinner			
	Bedtime			
Friday	Breakfast			
	Lunch			
	Dinner			
	Bedtime			
Saturday	Breakfast			
	Lunch			
	Dinner			
	Bedtime			

Blood Sugar Tracker

WEEK OF: _________________

Day	Time	Before	After	Notes
Sunday	Breakfast Lunch Dinner Bedtime			
Monday	Breakfast Lunch Dinner Bedtime			
Tuesday	Breakfast Lunch Dinner Bedtime			
Wednesday	Breakfast Lunch Dinner Bedtime			
Thursday	Breakfast Lunch Dinner Bedtime			
Friday	Breakfast Lunch Dinner Bedtime			
Saturday	Breakfast Lunch Dinner Bedtime			

Blood Sugar Tracker

WEEK OF: _____________________

	Time	Before	After	Notes
Sunday	Breakfast			
	Lunch			
	Dinner			
	Bedtime			
Monday	Breakfast			
	Lunch			
	Dinner			
	Bedtime			
Tuesday	Breakfast			
	Lunch			
	Dinner			
	Bedtime			
Wednesday	Breakfast			
	Lunch			
	Dinner			
	Bedtime			
Thursday	Breakfast			
	Lunch			
	Dinner			
	Bedtime			
Friday	Breakfast			
	Lunch			
	Dinner			
	Bedtime			
Saturday	Breakfast			
	Lunch			
	Dinner			
	Bedtime			

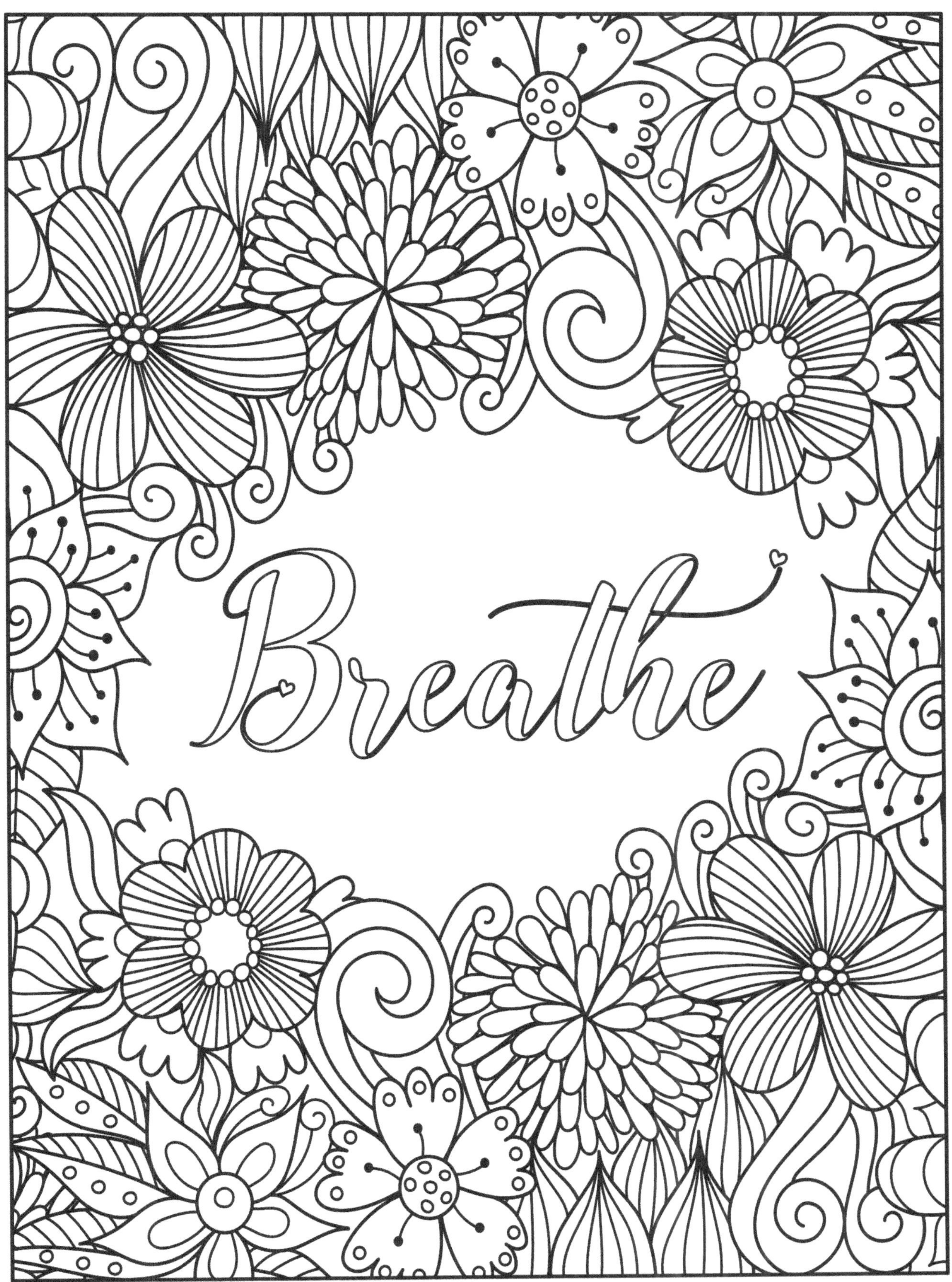

Breathe

Blood Sugar Tracker

WEEK OF: _______________________

Day	Time	Before	After	Notes
Sunday	Breakfast Lunch Dinner Bedtime			
Monday	Breakfast Lunch Dinner Bedtime			
Tuesday	Breakfast Lunch Dinner Bedtime			
Wednesday	Breakfast Lunch Dinner Bedtime			
Thursday	Breakfast Lunch Dinner Bedtime			
Friday	Breakfast Lunch Dinner Bedtime			
Saturday	Breakfast Lunch Dinner Bedtime			

Blood Sugar Tracker

WEEK OF: _______________________

<table>
<tr><td></td><td>Time</td><td>Before</td><td>After</td><td>Notes</td></tr>
<tr><td rowspan="4">Sunday</td><td>Breakfast</td><td></td><td></td><td></td></tr>
<tr><td>Lunch</td><td></td><td></td><td></td></tr>
<tr><td>Dinner</td><td></td><td></td><td></td></tr>
<tr><td>Bedtime</td><td></td><td></td><td></td></tr>
<tr><td rowspan="4">Monday</td><td>Breakfast</td><td></td><td></td><td></td></tr>
<tr><td>Lunch</td><td></td><td></td><td></td></tr>
<tr><td>Dinner</td><td></td><td></td><td></td></tr>
<tr><td>Bedtime</td><td></td><td></td><td></td></tr>
<tr><td rowspan="4">Tuesday</td><td>Breakfast</td><td></td><td></td><td></td></tr>
<tr><td>Lunch</td><td></td><td></td><td></td></tr>
<tr><td>Dinner</td><td></td><td></td><td></td></tr>
<tr><td>Bedtime</td><td></td><td></td><td></td></tr>
<tr><td rowspan="4">Wednesday</td><td>Breakfast</td><td></td><td></td><td></td></tr>
<tr><td>Lunch</td><td></td><td></td><td></td></tr>
<tr><td>Dinner</td><td></td><td></td><td></td></tr>
<tr><td>Bedtime</td><td></td><td></td><td></td></tr>
<tr><td rowspan="4">Thursday</td><td>Breakfast</td><td></td><td></td><td></td></tr>
<tr><td>Lunch</td><td></td><td></td><td></td></tr>
<tr><td>Dinner</td><td></td><td></td><td></td></tr>
<tr><td>Bedtime</td><td></td><td></td><td></td></tr>
<tr><td rowspan="4">Friday</td><td>Breakfast</td><td></td><td></td><td></td></tr>
<tr><td>Lunch</td><td></td><td></td><td></td></tr>
<tr><td>Dinner</td><td></td><td></td><td></td></tr>
<tr><td>Bedtime</td><td></td><td></td><td></td></tr>
<tr><td rowspan="4">Saturday</td><td>Breakfast</td><td></td><td></td><td></td></tr>
<tr><td>Lunch</td><td></td><td></td><td></td></tr>
<tr><td>Dinner</td><td></td><td></td><td></td></tr>
<tr><td>Bedtime</td><td></td><td></td><td></td></tr>
</table>

Blood Sugar Tracker

WEEK OF: _______________

BREAKFAST			
LUNCH			
DINNER			
BEDTIME			
BREAKFAST			
LUNCH			
DINNER			
BEDTIME			
BREAKFAST			
LUNCH			
DINNER			
BEDTIME			
BREAKFAST			
LUNCH			
DINNER			
BEDTIME			
BREAKFAST			
LUNCH			
DINNER			
BEDTIME			
BREAKFAST			
LUNCH			
DINNER			
BEDTIME			
BREAKFAST			
LUNCH			
DINNER			
BEDTIME			

Blood Sugar Tracker

WEEK OF: ________________________

	Time	Before	After	Notes
Sunday	Breakfast			
	Lunch			
	Dinner			
	Bedtime			
Monday	Breakfast			
	Lunch			
	Dinner			
	Bedtime			
Tuesday	Breakfast			
	Lunch			
	Dinner			
	Bedtime			
Wednesday	Breakfast			
	Lunch			
	Dinner			
	Bedtime			
Thursday	Breakfast			
	Lunch			
	Dinner			
	Bedtime			
Friday	Breakfast			
	Lunch			
	Dinner			
	Bedtime			
Saturday	Breakfast			
	Lunch			
	Dinner			
	Bedtime			

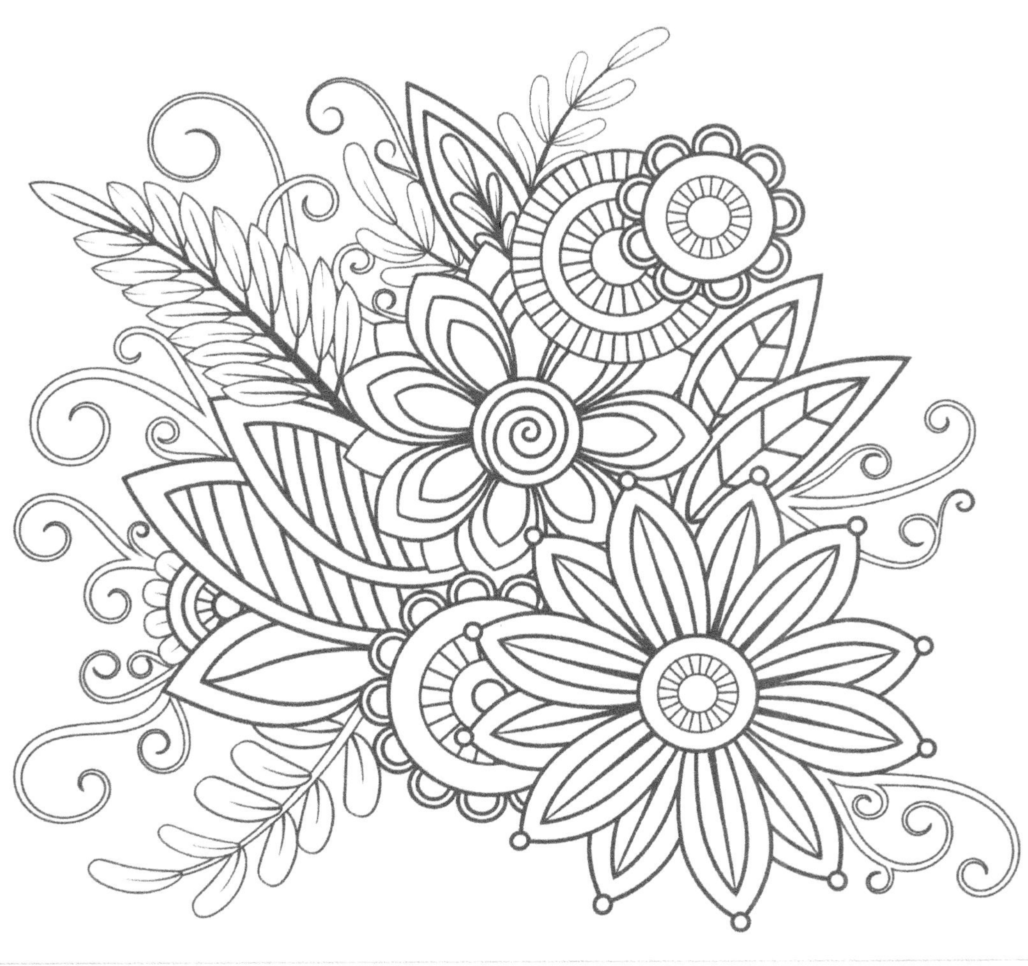

NOTES:

Blood Sugar Tracker

WEEK OF: _______________________

BREAKFAST
LUNCH
DINNER
BEDTIME

BREAKFAST
LUNCH
DINNER
BEDTIME

BREAKFAST
LUNCH
DINNER
BEDTIME

BREAKFAST
LUNCH
DINNER
BEDTIME

BREAKFAST
LUNCH
DINNER
BEDTIME

BREAKFAST
LUNCH
DINNER
BEDTIME

BREAKFAST
LUNCH
DINNER
BEDTIME

Blood Sugar Tracker

WEEK OF: _______________________

	Time	Before	After	Notes
Sunday	Breakfast			
	Lunch			
	Dinner			
	Bedtime			
Monday	Breakfast			
	Lunch			
	Dinner			
	Bedtime			
Tuesday	Breakfast			
	Lunch			
	Dinner			
	Bedtime			
Wednesday	Breakfast			
	Lunch			
	Dinner			
	Bedtime			
Thursday	Breakfast			
	Lunch			
	Dinner			
	Bedtime			
Friday	Breakfast			
	Lunch			
	Dinner			
	Bedtime			
Saturday	Breakfast			
	Lunch			
	Dinner			
	Bedtime			

Blood Sugar Tracker

WEEK OF: _________________

	TIME	BEFORE	AFTER	NOTES
SUNDAY	Breakfast Lunch Dinner Bedtime			
MONDAY	Breakfast Lunch Dinner Bedtime			
TUESDAY	Breakfast Lunch Dinner Bedtime			
WEDNESDAY	Breakfast Lunch Dinner Bedtime			
THURSDAY	Breakfast Lunch Dinner Bedtime			
FRIDAY	Breakfast Lunch Dinner Bedtime			
SATURDAY	Breakfast Lunch Dinner Bedtime			

Blood Sugar Tracker

WEEK OF: _________________________

	Time	Before	After	Notes
Sunday	Breakfast			
	Lunch			
	Dinner			
	Bedtime			
Monday	Breakfast			
	Lunch			
	Dinner			
	Bedtime			
Tuesday	Breakfast			
	Lunch			
	Dinner			
	Bedtime			
Wednesday	Breakfast			
	Lunch			
	Dinner			
	Bedtime			
Thursday	Breakfast			
	Lunch			
	Dinner			
	Bedtime			
Friday	Breakfast			
	Lunch			
	Dinner			
	Bedtime			
Saturday	Breakfast			
	Lunch			
	Dinner			
	Bedtime			

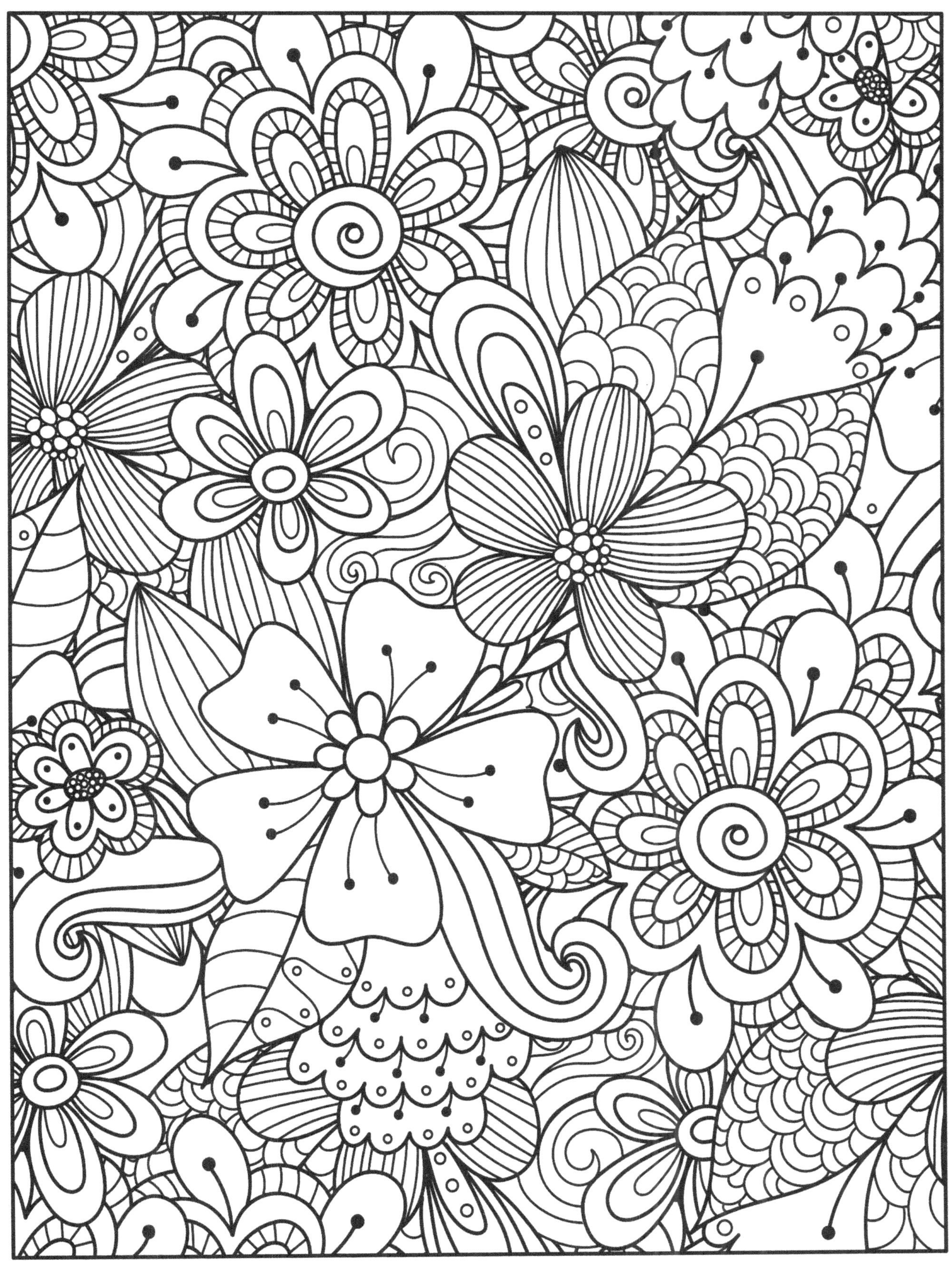

Blood Sugar Tracker

WEEK OF: _________________

	Time	Before	After	Notes
Sunday	Breakfast Lunch Dinner Bedtime			
Monday	Breakfast Lunch Dinner Bedtime			
Tuesday	Breakfast Lunch Dinner Bedtime			
Wednesday	Breakfast Lunch Dinner Bedtime			
Thursday	Breakfast Lunch Dinner Bedtime			
Friday	Breakfast Lunch Dinner Bedtime			
Saturday	Breakfast Lunch Dinner Bedtime			

Blood Sugar Tracker

WEEK OF: _______________________

Time	Before	After	Notes

Sunday

Time	Before	After	Notes
Breakfast			
Lunch			
Dinner			
Bedtime			

Monday

Breakfast			
Lunch			
Dinner			
Bedtime			

Tuesday

Breakfast			
Lunch			
Dinner			
Bedtime			

Wednesday

Breakfast			
Lunch			
Dinner			
Bedtime			

Thursday

Breakfast			
Lunch			
Dinner			
Bedtime			

Friday

Breakfast			
Lunch			
Dinner			
Bedtime			

Saturday

Breakfast			
Lunch			
Dinner			
Bedtime			

Blood Sugar Tracker

WEEK OF: ___________________

Breakfast			
Lunch			
Dinner			
Bedtime			
Breakfast			
Lunch			
Dinner			
Bedtime			
Breakfast			
Lunch			
Dinner			
Bedtime			
Breakfast			
Lunch			
Dinner			
Bedtime			
Breakfast			
Lunch			
Dinner			
Bedtime			
Breakfast			
Lunch			
Dinner			
Bedtime			
Breakfast			
Lunch			
Dinner			
Bedtime			

Blood Sugar Tracker

WEEK OF: _______________________

	Time	Before	After	Notes
Sunday	Breakfast Lunch Dinner Bedtime			
Monday	Breakfast Lunch Dinner Bedtime			
Tuesday	Breakfast Lunch Dinner Bedtime			
Wednesday	Breakfast Lunch Dinner Bedtime			
Thursday	Breakfast Lunch Dinner Bedtime			
Friday	Breakfast Lunch Dinner Bedtime			
Saturday	Breakfast Lunch Dinner Bedtime			

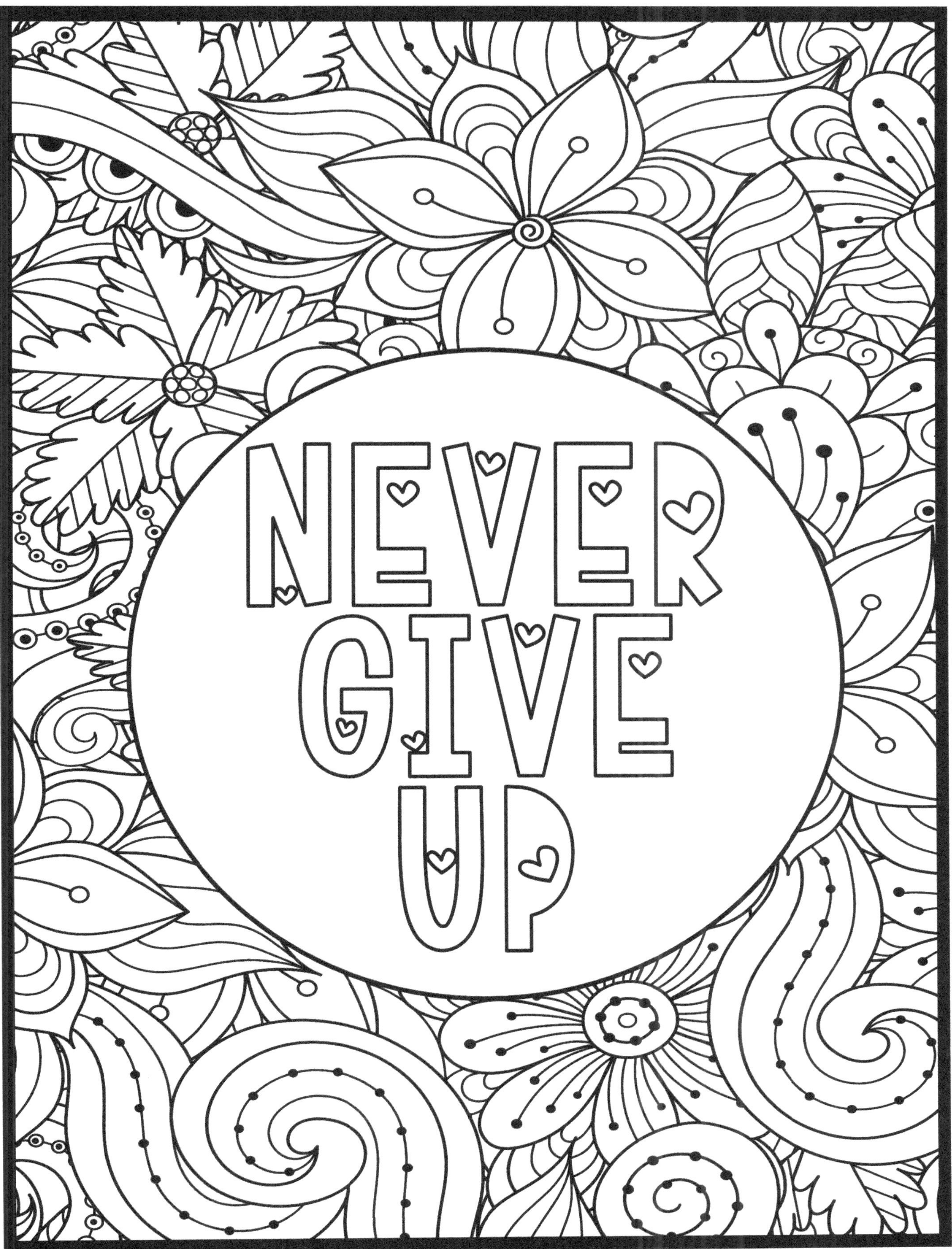

NEVER
GIVE
UP

Blood Sugar Tracker

Time			
Breakfast			
Lunch			
Dinner			
Bedtime			
Breakfast			
Lunch			
Dinner			
Bedtime			
Breakfast			
Lunch			
Dinner			
Bedtime			
Breakfast			
Lunch			
Dinner			
Bedtime			
Breakfast			
Lunch			
Dinner			
Bedtime			
Breakfast			
Lunch			
Dinner			
Bedtime			
Breakfast			
Lunch			
Dinner			
Bedtime			

BLOOD SUGAR TRACKER

WEEK OF: ______________________

Day	Time	Before	After	Notes
Sunday	Breakfast			
	Lunch			
	Dinner			
	Bedtime			
Monday	Breakfast			
	Lunch			
	Dinner			
	Bedtime			
Tuesday	Breakfast			
	Lunch			
	Dinner			
	Bedtime			
Wednesday	Breakfast			
	Lunch			
	Dinner			
	Bedtime			
Thursday	Breakfast			
	Lunch			
	Dinner			
	Bedtime			
Friday	Breakfast			
	Lunch			
	Dinner			
	Bedtime			
Saturday	Breakfast			
	Lunch			
	Dinner			
	Bedtime			

Blood Sugar Tracker

WEEK OF: ___________________

	Times	Before	After	Notes
Sunday	Breakfast Lunch Dinner Bedtime			
Monday	Breakfast Lunch Dinner Bedtime			
Tuesday	Breakfast Lunch Dinner Bedtime			
Wednesday	Breakfast Lunch Dinner Bedtime			
Thursday	Breakfast Lunch Dinner Bedtime			
Friday	Breakfast Lunch Dinner Bedtime			
Saturday	Breakfast Lunch Dinner Bedtime			

Blood Sugar Tracker

WEEK OF: _______________________

	Time	Before	After	Notes
Sunday	Breakfast			
	Lunch			
	Dinner			
	Bedtime			
Monday	Breakfast			
	Lunch			
	Dinner			
	Bedtime			
Tuesday	Breakfast			
	Lunch			
	Dinner			
	Bedtime			
Wednesday	Breakfast			
	Lunch			
	Dinner			
	Bedtime			
Thursday	Breakfast			
	Lunch			
	Dinner			
	Bedtime			
Friday	Breakfast			
	Lunch			
	Dinner			
	Bedtime			
Saturday	Breakfast			
	Lunch			
	Dinner			
	Bedtime			

NOTES:

Blood Sugar Tracker

WEEK OF: _________________

<table>
<tr><td></td><td>Time</td><td>Before</td><td>After</td><td>Notes</td></tr>
<tr><td rowspan="4">Sunday</td><td>Breakfast</td><td></td><td></td><td></td></tr>
<tr><td>Lunch</td><td></td><td></td><td></td></tr>
<tr><td>Dinner</td><td></td><td></td><td></td></tr>
<tr><td>Bedtime</td><td></td><td></td><td></td></tr>
<tr><td rowspan="4">Monday</td><td>Breakfast</td><td></td><td></td><td></td></tr>
<tr><td>Lunch</td><td></td><td></td><td></td></tr>
<tr><td>Dinner</td><td></td><td></td><td></td></tr>
<tr><td>Bedtime</td><td></td><td></td><td></td></tr>
<tr><td rowspan="4">Tuesday</td><td>Breakfast</td><td></td><td></td><td></td></tr>
<tr><td>Lunch</td><td></td><td></td><td></td></tr>
<tr><td>Dinner</td><td></td><td></td><td></td></tr>
<tr><td>Bedtime</td><td></td><td></td><td></td></tr>
<tr><td rowspan="4">Wednesday</td><td>Breakfast</td><td></td><td></td><td></td></tr>
<tr><td>Lunch</td><td></td><td></td><td></td></tr>
<tr><td>Dinner</td><td></td><td></td><td></td></tr>
<tr><td>Bedtime</td><td></td><td></td><td></td></tr>
<tr><td rowspan="4">Thursday</td><td>Breakfast</td><td></td><td></td><td></td></tr>
<tr><td>Lunch</td><td></td><td></td><td></td></tr>
<tr><td>Dinner</td><td></td><td></td><td></td></tr>
<tr><td>Bedtime</td><td></td><td></td><td></td></tr>
<tr><td rowspan="4">Friday</td><td>Breakfast</td><td></td><td></td><td></td></tr>
<tr><td>Lunch</td><td></td><td></td><td></td></tr>
<tr><td>Dinner</td><td></td><td></td><td></td></tr>
<tr><td>Bedtime</td><td></td><td></td><td></td></tr>
<tr><td rowspan="4">Saturday</td><td>Breakfast</td><td></td><td></td><td></td></tr>
<tr><td>Lunch</td><td></td><td></td><td></td></tr>
<tr><td>Dinner</td><td></td><td></td><td></td></tr>
<tr><td>Bedtime</td><td></td><td></td><td></td></tr>
</table>

BLOOD SUGAR TRACKER

WEEK OF: _______________________

	Time	Before	After	Notes
Sunday	BREAKFAST			
	LUNCH			
	DINNER			
	BEDTIME			
Monday	BREAKFAST			
	LUNCH			
	DINNER			
	BEDTIME			
Tuesday	BREAKFAST			
	LUNCH			
	DINNER			
	BEDTIME			
Wednesday	BREAKFAST			
	LUNCH			
	DINNER			
	BEDTIME			
Thursday	BREAKFAST			
	LUNCH			
	DINNER			
	BEDTIME			
Friday	BREAKFAST			
	LUNCH			
	DINNER			
	BEDTIME			
Saturday	BREAKFAST			
	LUNCH			
	DINNER			
	BEDTIME			

Blood Sugar Tracker

	Time	Before	After	Notes
Monday	Breakfast			
	Lunch			
	Dinner			
	Bedtime			
Tuesday	Breakfast			
	Lunch			
	Dinner			
	Bedtime			
Wednesday	Breakfast			
	Lunch			
	Dinner			
	Bedtime			
Thursday	Breakfast			
	Lunch			
	Dinner			
	Bedtime			
Friday	Breakfast			
	Lunch			
	Dinner			
	Bedtime			
Saturday	Breakfast			
	Lunch			
	Dinner			
	Bedtime			
Sunday	Breakfast			
	Lunch			
	Dinner			
	Bedtime			

Blood Sugar Tracker

WEEK OF: ________________

	Time	Before	After	Notes
Sunday	Breakfast			
	Lunch			
	Dinner			
	Bedtime			
Monday	Breakfast			
	Lunch			
	Dinner			
	Bedtime			
Tuesday	Breakfast			
	Lunch			
	Dinner			
	Bedtime			
Wednesday	Breakfast			
	Lunch			
	Dinner			
	Bedtime			
Thursday	Breakfast			
	Lunch			
	Dinner			
	Bedtime			
Friday	Breakfast			
	Lunch			
	Dinner			
	Bedtime			
Saturday	Breakfast			
	Lunch			
	Dinner			
	Bedtime			

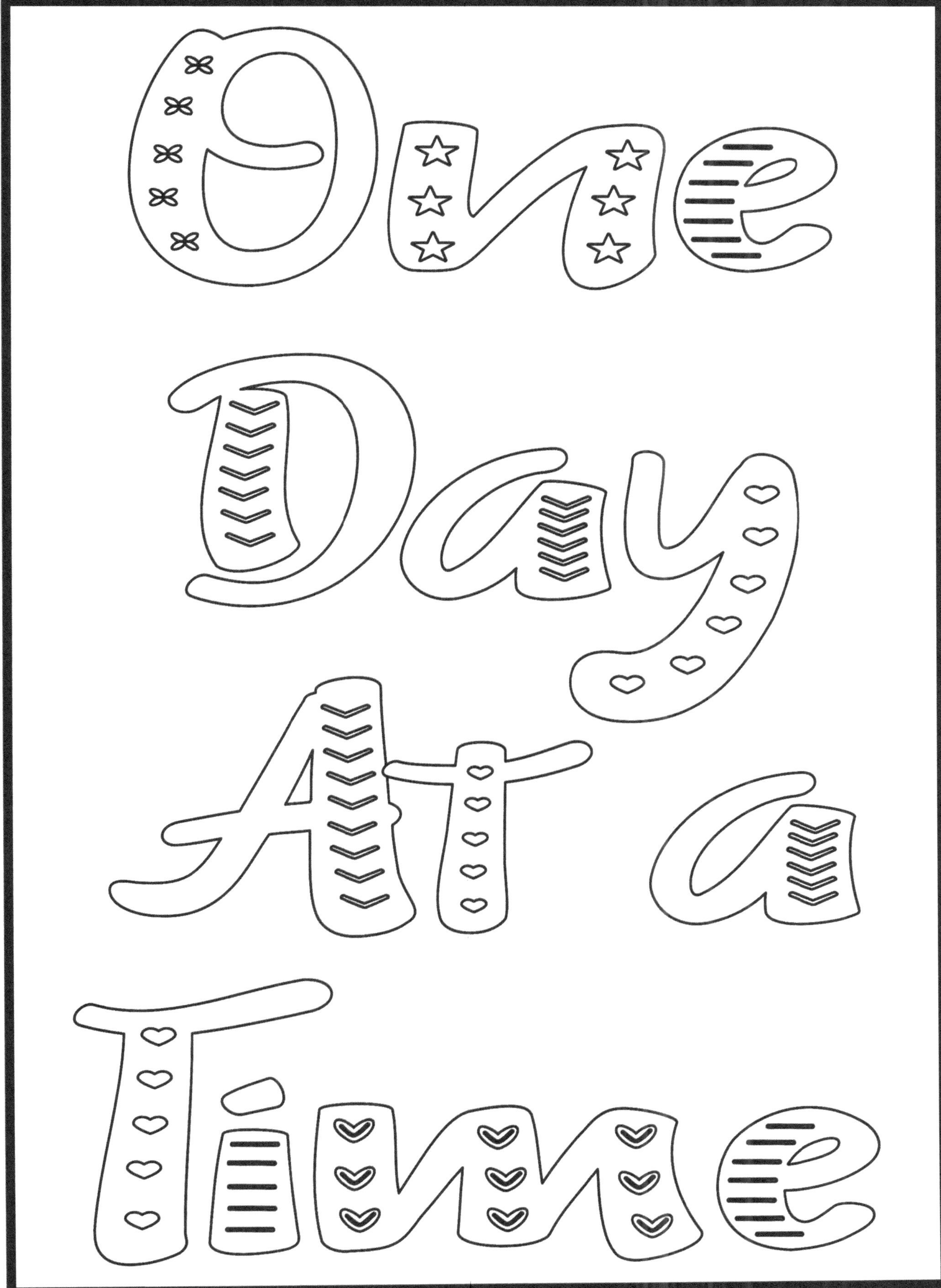

One
Day
At a
Time

Blood Sugar Tracker

WEEK OF: _______________

		Before	After	Notes
Sunday	Breakfast			
	Lunch			
	Dinner			
	Bedtime			
Monday	Breakfast			
	Lunch			
	Dinner			
	Bedtime			
Tuesday	Breakfast			
	Lunch			
	Dinner			
	Bedtime			
Wednesday	Breakfast			
	Lunch			
	Dinner			
	Bedtime			
Thursday	Breakfast			
	Lunch			
	Dinner			
	Bedtime			
Friday	Breakfast			
	Lunch			
	Dinner			
	Bedtime			
Saturday	Breakfast			
	Lunch			
	Dinner			
	Bedtime			

Blood Sugar Tracker

WEEK OF: ________________

	Time	Before	After	Notes
Sunday	Breakfast Lunch Dinner Bedtime			
Monday	Breakfast Lunch Dinner Bedtime			
Tuesday	Breakfast Lunch Dinner Bedtime			
Wednesday	Breakfast Lunch Dinner Bedtime			
Thursday	Breakfast Lunch Dinner Bedtime			
Friday	Breakfast Lunch Dinner Bedtime			
Saturday	Breakfast Lunch Dinner Bedtime			

Blood Sugar Tracker

WEEK OF: _______________________

	Time	Before	After	Notes
Sunday	Breakfast Lunch Dinner Bedtime			
Monday	Breakfast Lunch Dinner Bedtime			
Tuesday	Breakfast Lunch Dinner Bedtime			
Wednesday	Breakfast Lunch Dinner Bedtime			
Thursday	Breakfast Lunch Dinner Bedtime			
Friday	Breakfast Lunch Dinner Bedtime			
Saturday	Breakfast Lunch Dinner Bedtime			

Blood Sugar Tracker

WEEK OF: _______________________

	Time	Before	After	Notes
Sunday	Breakfast			
	Lunch			
	Dinner			
	Bedtime			
Monday	Breakfast			
	Lunch			
	Dinner			
	Bedtime			
Tuesday	Breakfast			
	Lunch			
	Dinner			
	Bedtime			
Wednesday	Breakfast			
	Lunch			
	Dinner			
	Bedtime			
Thursday	Breakfast			
	Lunch			
	Dinner			
	Bedtime			
Friday	Breakfast			
	Lunch			
	Dinner			
	Bedtime			
Saturday	Breakfast			
	Lunch			
	Dinner			
	Bedtime			

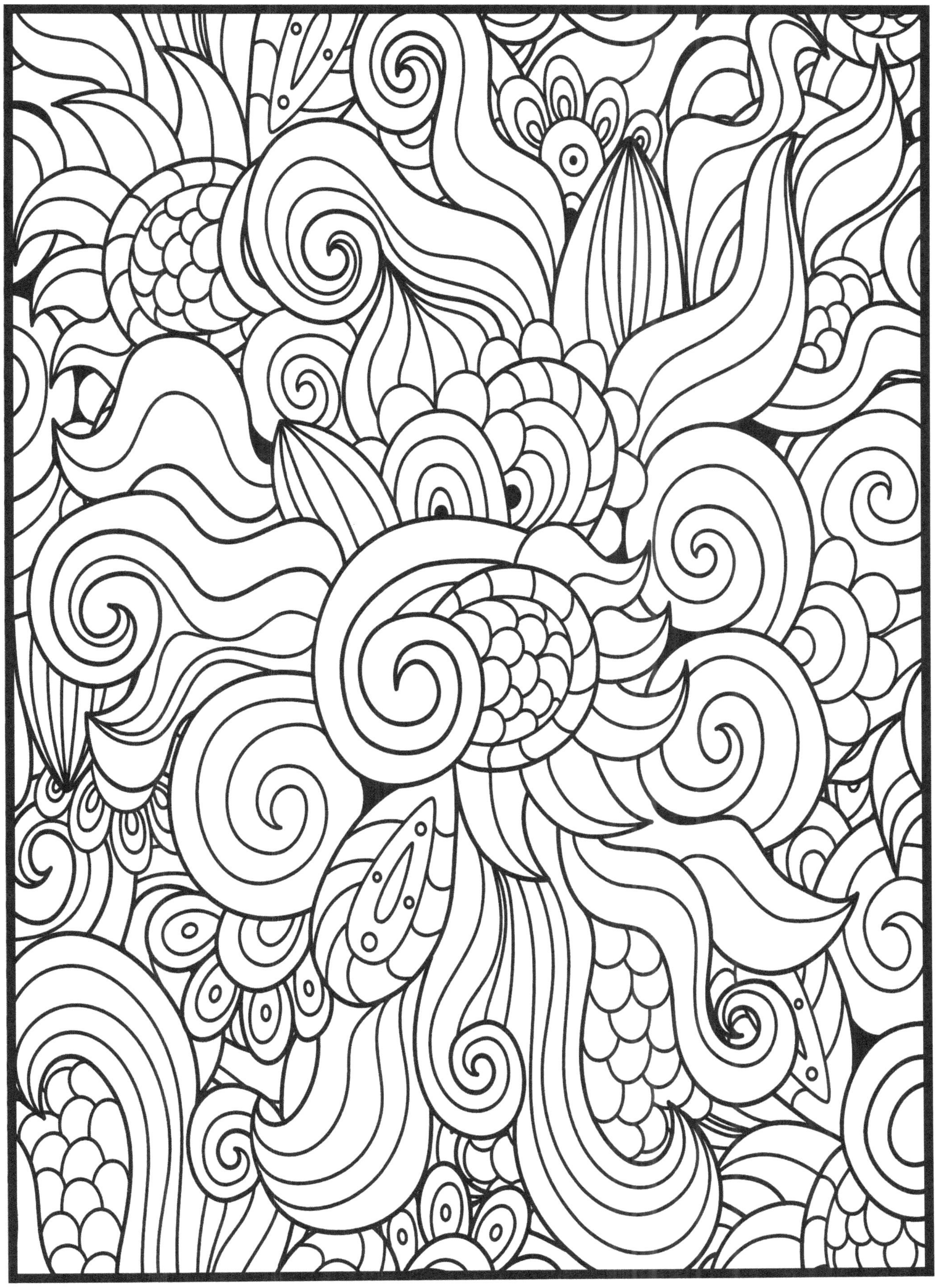

Blood Sugar Tracker

WEEK OF: ________________

	Time	Before	After	Notes
Sunday	Breakfast			
	Lunch			
	Dinner			
	Bedtime			
Monday	Breakfast			
	Lunch			
	Dinner			
	Bedtime			
Tuesday	Breakfast			
	Lunch			
	Dinner			
	Bedtime			
Wednesday	Breakfast			
	Lunch			
	Dinner			
	Bedtime			
Thursday	Breakfast			
	Lunch			
	Dinner			
	Bedtime			
Friday	Breakfast			
	Lunch			
	Dinner			
	Bedtime			
Saturday	Breakfast			
	Lunch			
	Dinner			
	Bedtime			

BLOOD SUGAR TRACKER

WEEK OF: _________________

	Time	Before	After	Notes
Sunday	BREAKFAST			
	LUNCH			
	DINNER			
	BEDTIME			
Monday	BREAKFAST			
	LUNCH			
	DINNER			
	BEDTIME			
Tuesday	BREAKFAST			
	LUNCH			
	DINNER			
	BEDTIME			
Wednesday	BREAKFAST			
	LUNCH			
	DINNER			
	BEDTIME			
Thursday	BREAKFAST			
	LUNCH			
	DINNER			
	BEDTIME			
Friday	BREAKFAST			
	LUNCH			
	DINNER			
	BEDTIME			
Saturday	BREAKFAST			
	LUNCH			
	DINNER			
	BEDTIME			

Blood Sugar Tracker

WEEK OF: _______________________

Breakfast Lunch Dinner Bedtime			
Breakfast Lunch Dinner Bedtime			
Breakfast Lunch Dinner Bedtime			
Breakfast Lunch Dinner Bedtime			
Breakfast Lunch Dinner Bedtime			
Breakfast Lunch Dinner Bedtime			
Breakfast Lunch Dinner Bedtime			

Blood Sugar Tracker

WEEK OF: ______________________

	Time	Before	After	Notes
Sunday	Breakfast			
	Lunch			
	Dinner			
	Bedtime			
Monday	Breakfast			
	Lunch			
	Dinner			
	Bedtime			
Tuesday	Breakfast			
	Lunch			
	Dinner			
	Bedtime			
Wednesday	Breakfast			
	Lunch			
	Dinner			
	Bedtime			
Thursday	Breakfast			
	Lunch			
	Dinner			
	Bedtime			
Friday	Breakfast			
	Lunch			
	Dinner			
	Bedtime			
Saturday	Breakfast			
	Lunch			
	Dinner			
	Bedtime			

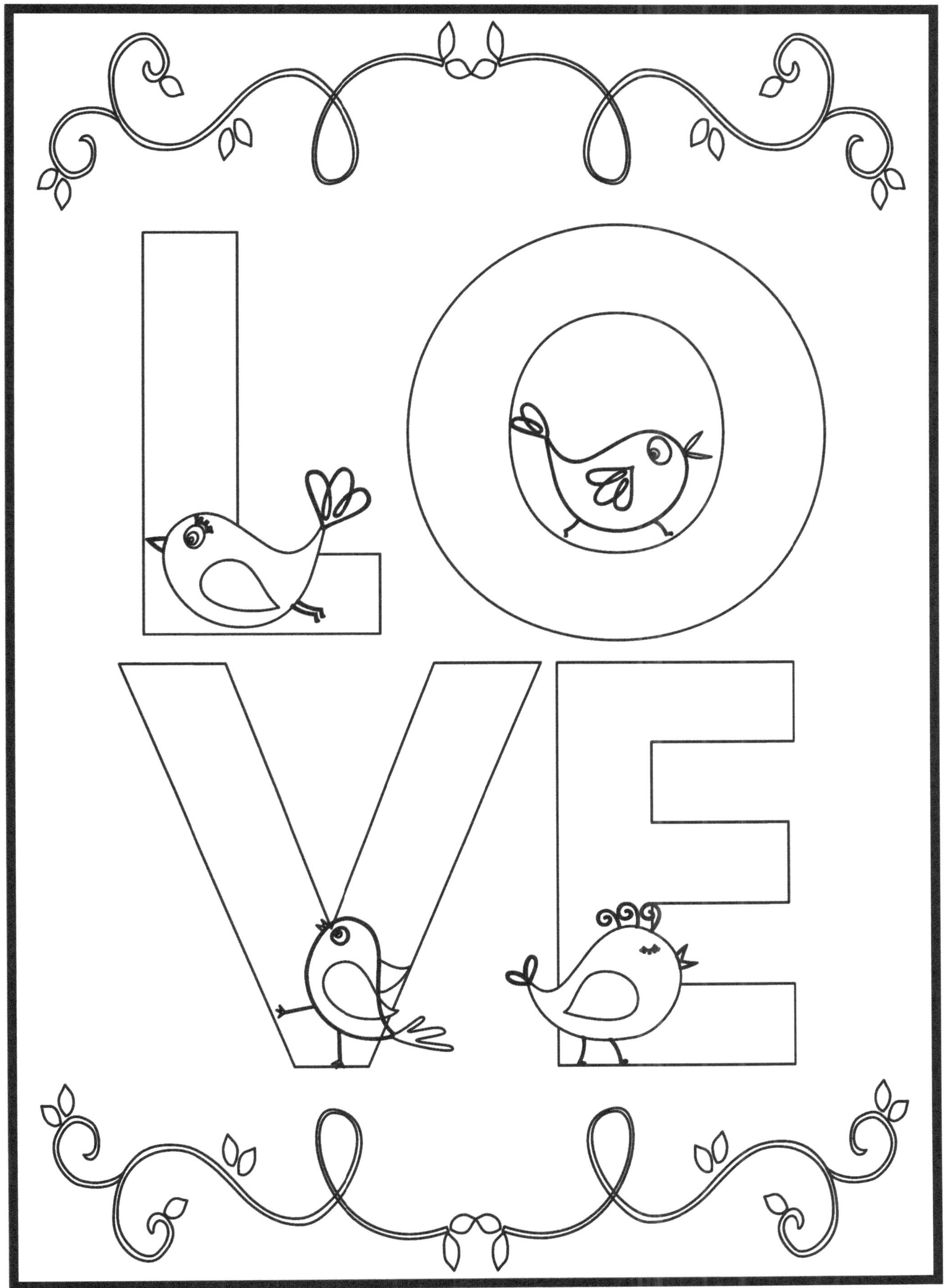

Blood Sugar Tracker

WEEK OF: ___________________

	BREAKFAST	LUNCH	DINNER	BEDTIME

BREAKFAST
LUNCH
DINNER
BEDTIME

BREAKFAST
LUNCH
DINNER
BEDTIME

BREAKFAST
LUNCH
DINNER
BEDTIME

BREAKFAST
LUNCH
DINNER
BEDTIME

BREAKFAST
LUNCH
DINNER
BEDTIME

BREAKFAST
LUNCH
DINNER
BEDTIME

BREAKFAST
LUNCH
DINNER
BEDTIME

Blood Sugar Tracker

WEEK OF: _______________________

	Time	Before	After	Notes
Sunday	Breakfast			
	Lunch			
	Dinner			
	Bedtime			
Monday	Breakfast			
	Lunch			
	Dinner			
	Bedtime			
Tuesday	Breakfast			
	Lunch			
	Dinner			
	Bedtime			
Wednesday	Breakfast			
	Lunch			
	Dinner			
	Bedtime			
Thursday	Breakfast			
	Lunch			
	Dinner			
	Bedtime			
Friday	Breakfast			
	Lunch			
	Dinner			
	Bedtime			
Saturday	Breakfast			
	Lunch			
	Dinner			
	Bedtime			

Blood Sugar Tracker

WEEK OF: _______________________

BREAKFAST
LUNCH
DINNER
BEDTIME

BREAKFAST
LUNCH
DINNER
BEDTIME

BREAKFAST
LUNCH
DINNER
BEDTIME

BREAKFAST
LUNCH
DINNER
BEDTIME

BREAKFAST
LUNCH
DINNER
BEDTIME

BREAKFAST
LUNCH
DINNER
BEDTIME

BREAKFAST
LUNCH
DINNER
BEDTIME

Blood Sugar Tracker

WEEK OF: ______________________

Time	Before	After	Notes
Breakfast			
Lunch			
Dinner			
Bedtime			
Breakfast			
Lunch			
Dinner			
Bedtime			
Breakfast			
Lunch			
Dinner			
Bedtime			
Breakfast			
Lunch			
Dinner			
Bedtime			
Breakfast			
Lunch			
Dinner			
Bedtime			
Breakfast			
Lunch			
Dinner			
Bedtime			
Breakfast			
Lunch			
Dinner			
Bedtime			

NOTES:

Blood Sugar Tracker

WEEK OF: _________________________

	Time	Before	After	Notes
	Breakfast Lunch Dinner Bedtime			
	Breakfast Lunch Dinner Bedtime			
	Breakfast Lunch Dinner Bedtime			
	Breakfast Lunch Dinner Bedtime			
	Breakfast Lunch Dinner Bedtime			
	Breakfast Lunch Dinner Bedtime			
	Breakfast Lunch Dinner Bedtime			

Blood Sugar Tracker

WEEK OF: _______________________

	Time	Before	After	Notes
Sunday	BREAKFAST LUNCH DINNER BEDTIME			
Monday	BREAKFAST LUNCH DINNER BEDTIME			
Tuesday	BREAKFAST LUNCH DINNER BEDTIME			
Wednesday	BREAKFAST LUNCH DINNER BEDTIME			
Thursday	BREAKFAST LUNCH DINNER BEDTIME			
Friday	BREAKFAST LUNCH DINNER BEDTIME			
Saturday	BREAKFAST LUNCH DINNER BEDTIME			

Blood Sugar Tracker

BREAKFAST			
LUNCH			
DINNER			
BEDTIME			
BREAKFAST			
LUNCH			
DINNER			
BEDTIME			
BREAKFAST			
LUNCH			
DINNER			
BEDTIME			
BREAKFAST			
LUNCH			
DINNER			
BEDTIME			
BREAKFAST			
LUNCH			
DINNER			
BEDTIME			
BREAKFAST			
LUNCH			
DINNER			
BEDTIME			
BREAKFAST			
LUNCH			
DINNER			
BEDTIME			

Blood Sugar Tracker

WEEK OF: ___________________

	Time	Before	After	Notes
Sunday	Breakfast			
	Lunch			
	Dinner			
	Bedtime			
Monday	Breakfast			
	Lunch			
	Dinner			
	Bedtime			
Tuesday	Breakfast			
	Lunch			
	Dinner			
	Bedtime			
Wednesday	Breakfast			
	Lunch			
	Dinner			
	Bedtime			
Thursday	Breakfast			
	Lunch			
	Dinner			
	Bedtime			
Friday	Breakfast			
	Lunch			
	Dinner			
	Bedtime			
Saturday	Breakfast			
	Lunch			
	Dinner			
	Bedtime			

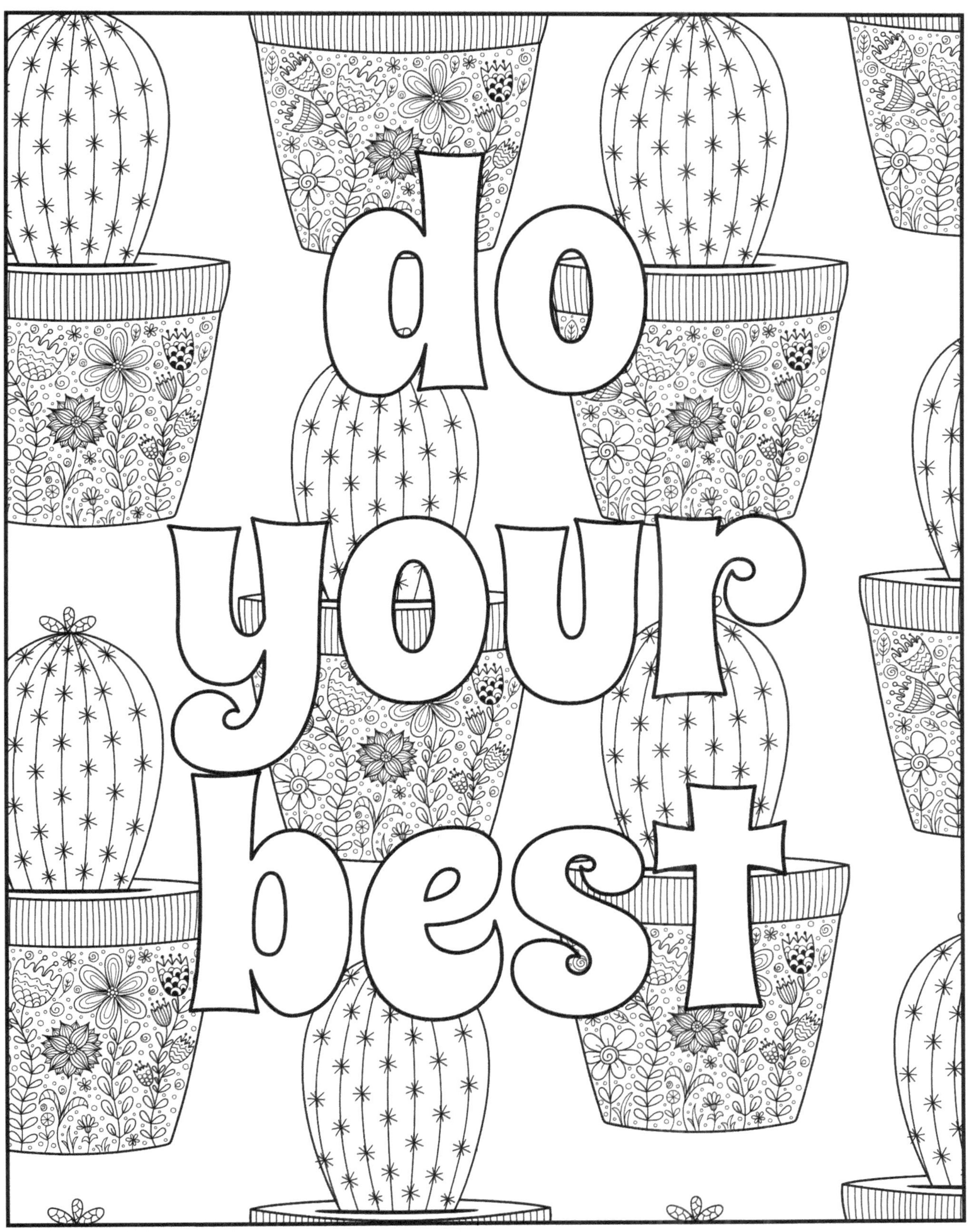

do
your
best

Blood Sugar Tracker

WEEK OF: _________________

Breakfast
Lunch
Dinner
Bedtime

Breakfast
Lunch
Dinner
Bedtime

Breakfast
Lunch
Dinner
Bedtime

Breakfast
Lunch
Dinner
Bedtime

Breakfast
Lunch
Dinner
Bedtime

Breakfast
Lunch
Dinner
Bedtime

Breakfast
Lunch
Dinner
Bedtime

Blood Sugar Tracker

WEEK OF: _______________

	Time	Before	After	Notes
Sunday	Breakfast Lunch Dinner Bedtime			
Monday	Breakfast Lunch Dinner Bedtime			
Tuesday	Breakfast Lunch Dinner Bedtime			
Wednesday	Breakfast Lunch Dinner Bedtime			
Thursday	Breakfast Lunch Dinner Bedtime			
Friday	Breakfast Lunch Dinner Bedtime			
Saturday	Breakfast Lunch Dinner Bedtime			

Blood Sugar Tracker

WEEK OF: _______________

BREAKFAST
LUNCH
DINNER
BEDTIME

BREAKFAST
LUNCH
DINNER
BEDTIME

BREAKFAST
LUNCH
DINNER
BEDTIME

BREAKFAST
LUNCH
DINNER
BEDTIME

BREAKFAST
LUNCH
DINNER
BEDTIME

BREAKFAST
LUNCH
DINNER
BEDTIME

BREAKFAST
LUNCH
DINNER
BEDTIME

BLOOD SUGAR TRACKER

WEEK OF: _________________

	Time	Before	After	Notes
Sunday	BREAKFAST			
	LUNCH			
	DINNER			
	BEDTIME			
Monday	BREAKFAST			
	LUNCH			
	DINNER			
	BEDTIME			
Tuesday	BREAKFAST			
	LUNCH			
	DINNER			
	BEDTIME			
Wednesday	BREAKFAST			
	LUNCH			
	DINNER			
	BEDTIME			
Thursday	BREAKFAST			
	LUNCH			
	DINNER			
	BEDTIME			
Friday	BREAKFAST			
	LUNCH			
	DINNER			
	BEDTIME			
Saturday	BREAKFAST			
	LUNCH			
	DINNER			
	BEDTIME			

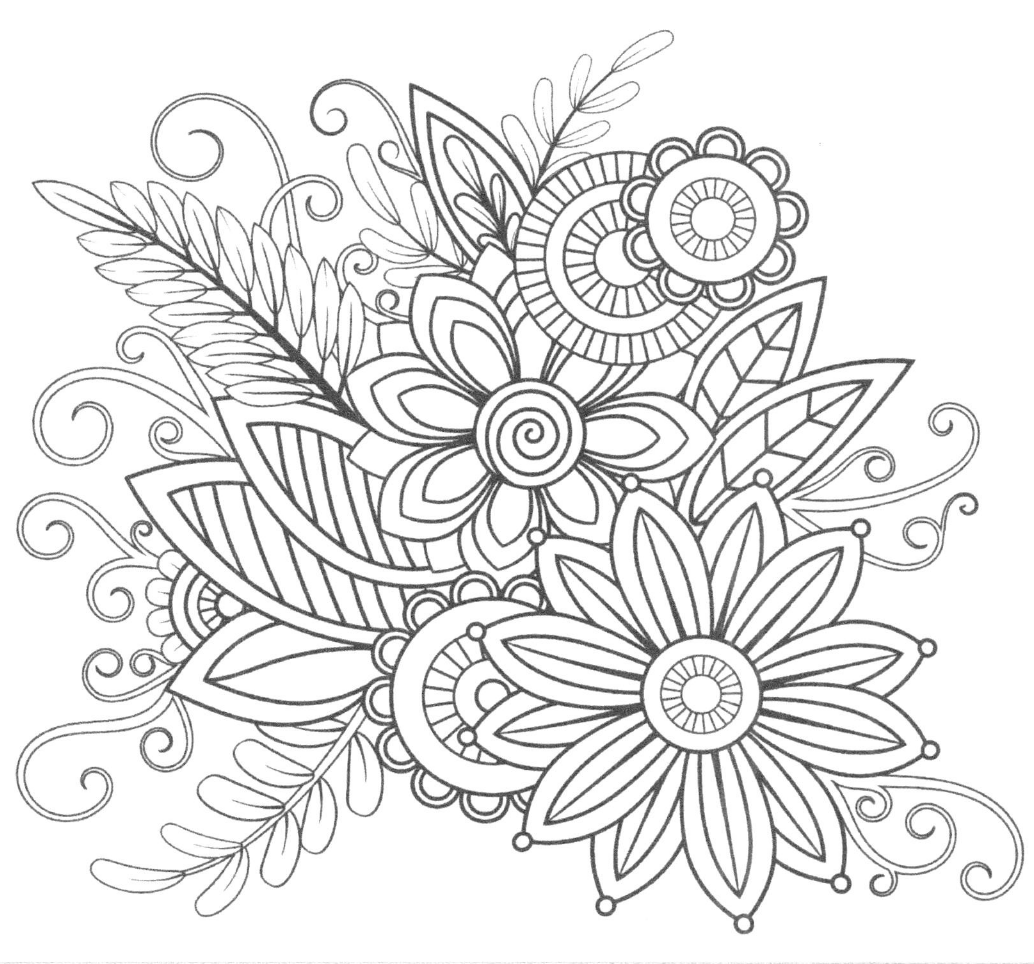

NOTES:

Blood Sugar Tracker

WEEK OF: _______________________

	Time	Before	After	Notes
Sunday	Breakfast			
	Lunch			
	Dinner			
	Bedtime			
Monday	Breakfast			
	Lunch			
	Dinner			
	Bedtime			
Tuesday	Breakfast			
	Lunch			
	Dinner			
	Bedtime			
Wednesday	Breakfast			
	Lunch			
	Dinner			
	Bedtime			
Thursday	Breakfast			
	Lunch			
	Dinner			
	Bedtime			
Friday	Breakfast			
	Lunch			
	Dinner			
	Bedtime			
Saturday	Breakfast			
	Lunch			
	Dinner			
	Bedtime			

Blood Sugar Tracker

WEEK OF: _______________________

	Time	Before	After	Notes
Sunday	Breakfast Lunch Dinner Bedtime			
Monday	Breakfast Lunch Dinner Bedtime			
Tuesday	Breakfast Lunch Dinner Bedtime			
Wednesday	Breakfast Lunch Dinner Bedtime			
Thursday	Breakfast Lunch Dinner Bedtime			
Friday	Breakfast Lunch Dinner Bedtime			
Saturday	Breakfast Lunch Dinner Bedtime			

Blood Sugar Tracker

WEEK OF: _______________________

BREAKFAST
LUNCH
DINNER
BEDTIME

BREAKFAST
LUNCH
DINNER
BEDTIME

BREAKFAST
LUNCH
DINNER
BEDTIME

BREAKFAST
LUNCH
DINNER
BEDTIME

BREAKFAST
LUNCH
DINNER
BEDTIME

BREAKFAST
LUNCH
DINNER
BEDTIME

BREAKFAST
LUNCH
DINNER
BEDTIME

Blood Sugar Tracker

WEEK OF: _______________________

	Time	Before	After	Notes
Sunday	Breakfast Lunch Dinner Bedtime			
Monday	Breakfast Lunch Dinner Bedtime			
Tuesday	Breakfast Lunch Dinner Bedtime			
Wednesday	Breakfast Lunch Dinner Bedtime			
Thursday	Breakfast Lunch Dinner Bedtime			
Friday	Breakfast Lunch Dinner Bedtime			
Saturday	Breakfast Lunch Dinner Bedtime			

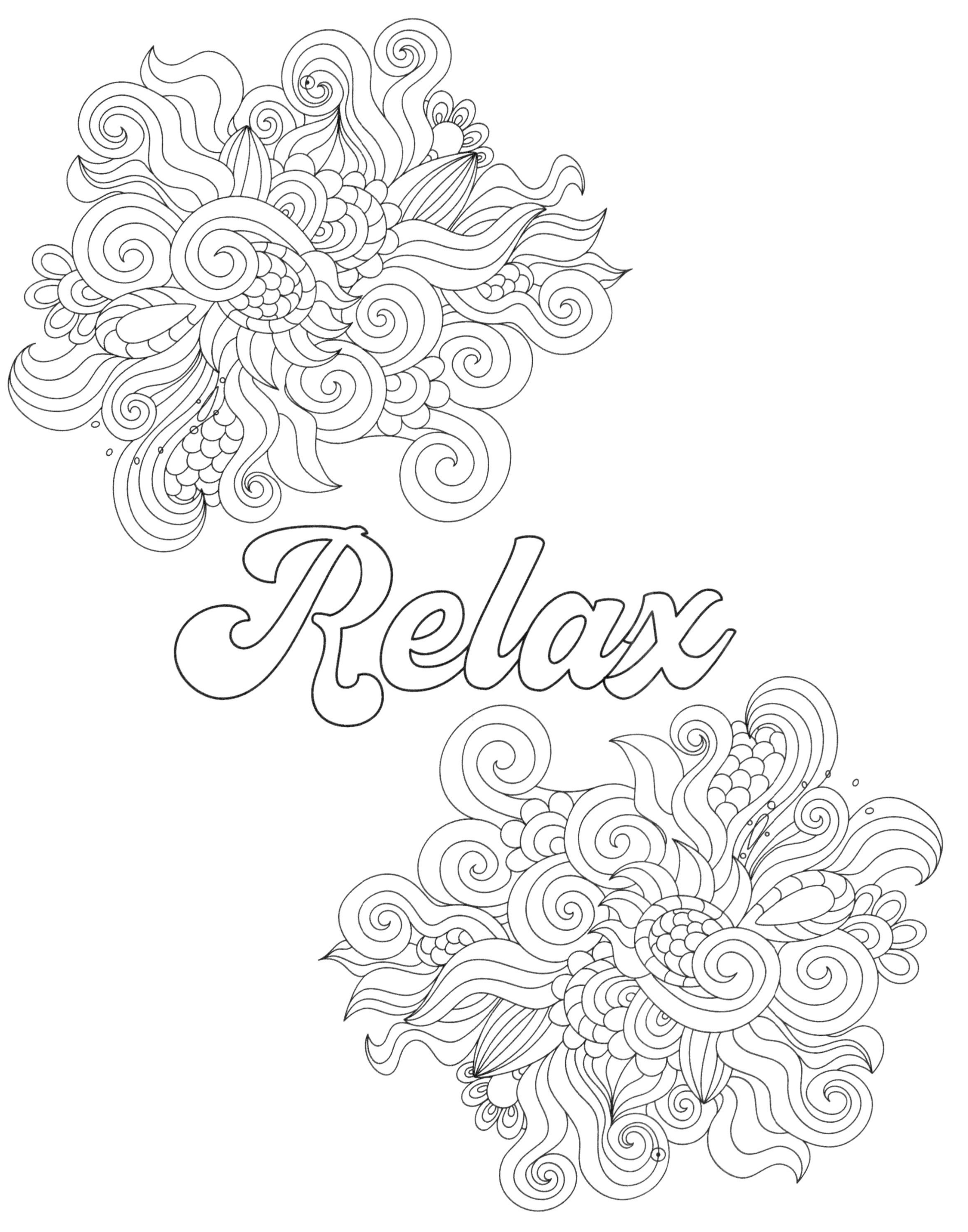
Relax

Blood Sugar Tracker

WEEK OF: _______________________

Breakfast
Lunch
Dinner
Bedtime

Breakfast
Lunch
Dinner
Bedtime

Breakfast
Lunch
Dinner
Bedtime

Breakfast
Lunch
Dinner
Bedtime

Breakfast
Lunch
Dinner
Bedtime

Breakfast
Lunch
Dinner
Bedtime

Breakfast
Lunch
Dinner
Bedtime

Blood Sugar Tracker

WEEK OF: _______________

	Time	Before	After	Notes
Sunday	Breakfast Lunch Dinner Bedtime			
Monday	Breakfast Lunch Dinner Bedtime			
Tuesday	Breakfast Lunch Dinner Bedtime			
Wednesday	Breakfast Lunch Dinner Bedtime			
Thursday	Breakfast Lunch Dinner Bedtime			
Friday	Breakfast Lunch Dinner Bedtime			
Saturday	Breakfast Lunch Dinner Bedtime			

Blood Sugar Tracker

BREAKFAST
LUNCH
DINNER
BEDTIME

BREAKFAST
LUNCH
DINNER
BEDTIME

BREAKFAST
LUNCH
DINNER
BEDTIME

BREAKFAST
LUNCH
DINNER
BEDTIME

BREAKFAST
LUNCH
DINNER
BEDTIME

BREAKFAST
LUNCH
DINNER
BEDTIME

BREAKFAST
LUNCH
DINNER
BEDTIME

Blood Sugar Tracker

WEEK OF: ___________________

	Time	Before	After	Notes
Sunday	Breakfast			
	Lunch			
	Dinner			
	Bedtime			
Monday	Breakfast			
	Lunch			
	Dinner			
	Bedtime			
Tuesday	Breakfast			
	Lunch			
	Dinner			
	Bedtime			
Wednesday	Breakfast			
	Lunch			
	Dinner			
	Bedtime			
Thursday	Breakfast			
	Lunch			
	Dinner			
	Bedtime			
Friday	Breakfast			
	Lunch			
	Dinner			
	Bedtime			
Saturday	Breakfast			
	Lunch			
	Dinner			
	Bedtime			

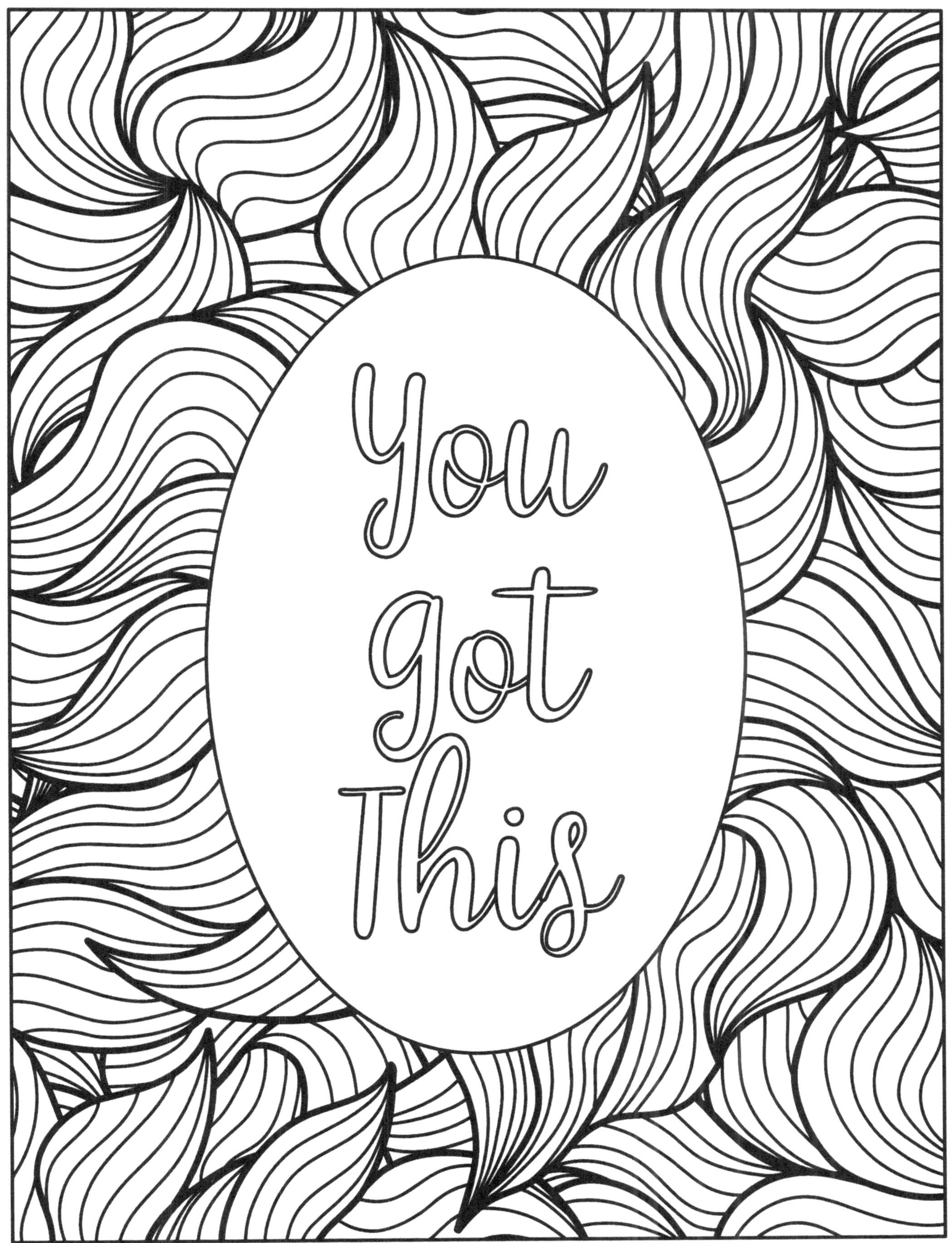

You
got
This

Blood Sugar Tracker

BREAKFAST
LUNCH
DINNER
BEDTIME

BREAKFAST
LUNCH
DINNER
BEDTIME

BREAKFAST
LUNCH
DINNER
BEDTIME

BREAKFAST
LUNCH
DINNER
BEDTIME

BREAKFAST
LUNCH
DINNER
BEDTIME

BREAKFAST
LUNCH
DINNER
BEDTIME

BREAKFAST
LUNCH
DINNER
BEDTIME

Blood Sugar Tracker

WEEK OF: _________________________

	Time	Before	After	Notes
Sunday	Breakfast Lunch Dinner Bedtime			
Monday	Breakfast Lunch Dinner Bedtime			
Tuesday	Breakfast Lunch Dinner Bedtime			
Wednesday	Breakfast Lunch Dinner Bedtime			
Thursday	Breakfast Lunch Dinner Bedtime			
Friday	Breakfast Lunch Dinner Bedtime			
Saturday	Breakfast Lunch Dinner Bedtime			

Blood Sugar Tracker

WEEK OF: _________________

BREAKFAST
LUNCH
DINNER
BEDTIME

BREAKFAST
LUNCH
DINNER
BEDTIME

BREAKFAST
LUNCH
DINNER
BEDTIME

BREAKFAST
LUNCH
DINNER
BEDTIME

BREAKFAST
LUNCH
DINNER
BEDTIME

BREAKFAST
LUNCH
DINNER
BEDTIME

BREAKFAST
LUNCH
DINNER
BEDTIME

Blood Sugar Tracker

WEEK OF: ________________

	Time	Before	After	Notes
Sunday	Breakfast Lunch Dinner Bedtime			
Monday	Breakfast Lunch Dinner Bedtime			
Tuesday	Breakfast Lunch Dinner Bedtime			
Wednesday	Breakfast Lunch Dinner Bedtime			
Thursday	Breakfast Lunch Dinner Bedtime			
Friday	Breakfast Lunch Dinner Bedtime			
Saturday	Breakfast Lunch Dinner Bedtime			

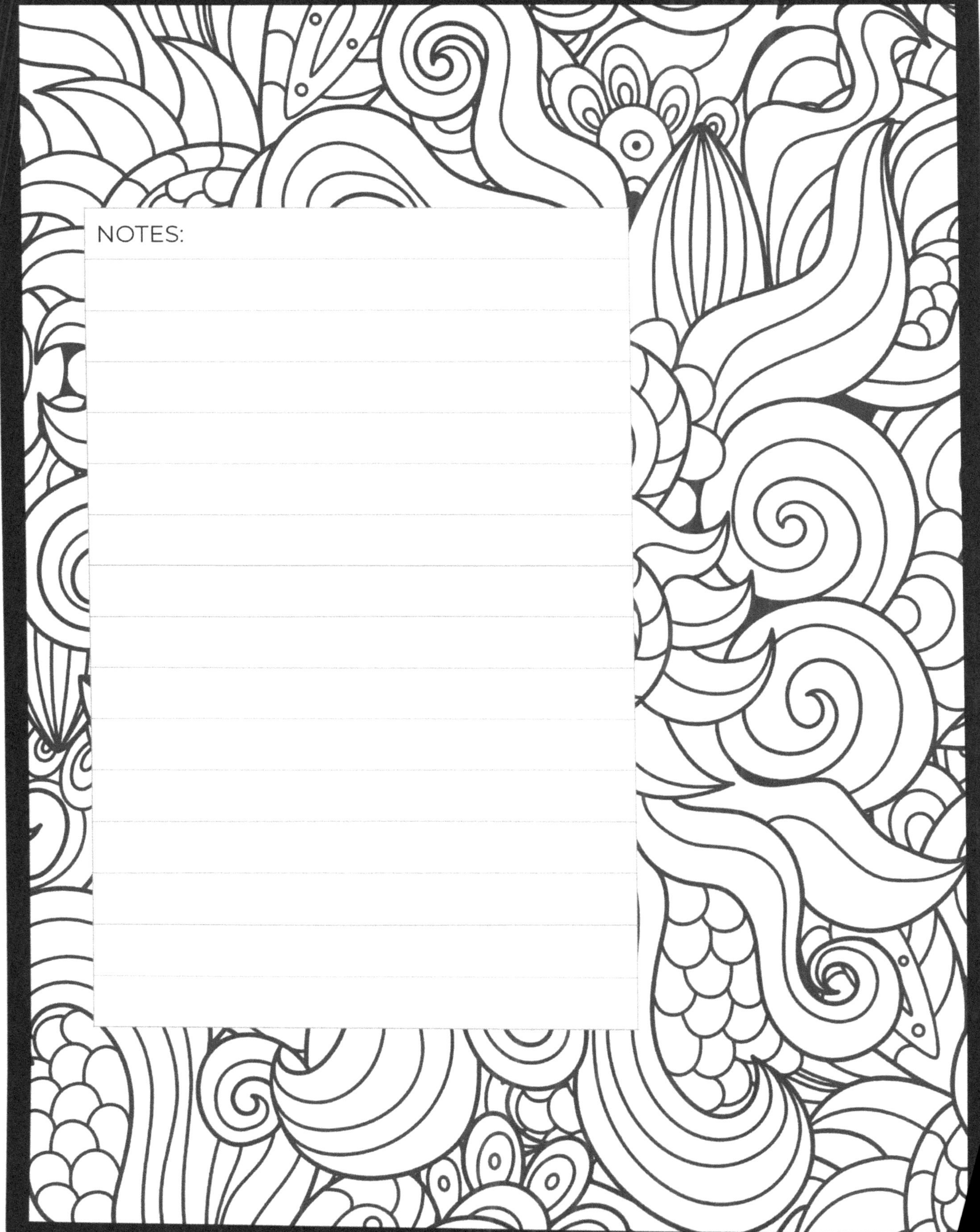

NOTES:

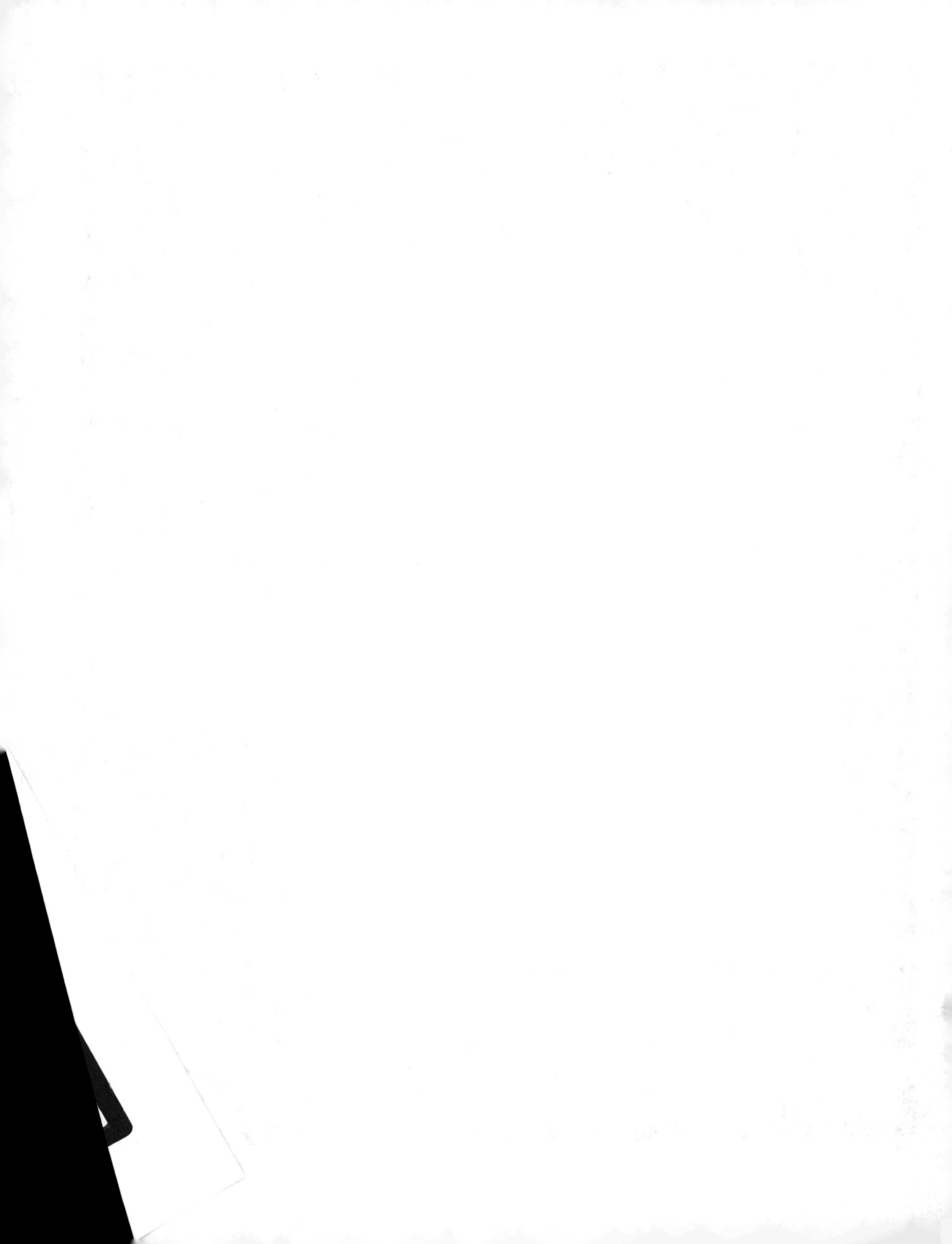